HANG toughF

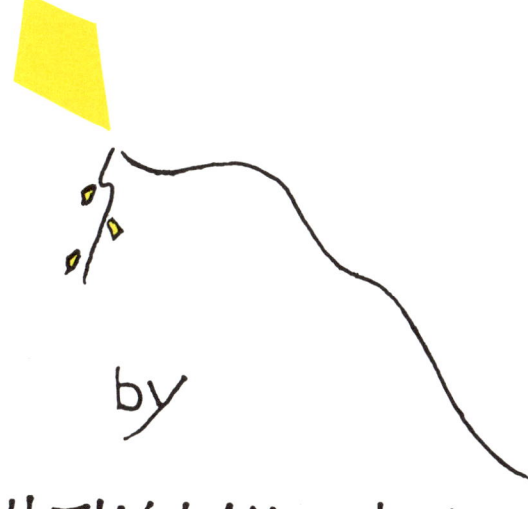

by

MATTHEW LANCASTER

paulist press • new york • mahwah

Thanks to Pamela Huffman for cover and additional interior art.

Copyright © 1983, 1985 by Jon W. and Martha R. Lancaster

All rights reserved. No part of this book may be reproduced or transmitted in any form, or by any means, electronic or mechanical including photocopying, recording or by any information storage and retrieval system, without permission in writing from the Publisher.

Library of Congress
Catalog Card Number: 85-60305

ISBN: 0-8091-2696-6

Published by Paulist Press
997 Macarthur Boulevard
Mahwah, New Jersey 07430

Printed and bound in the United States of America

to All People with cancer

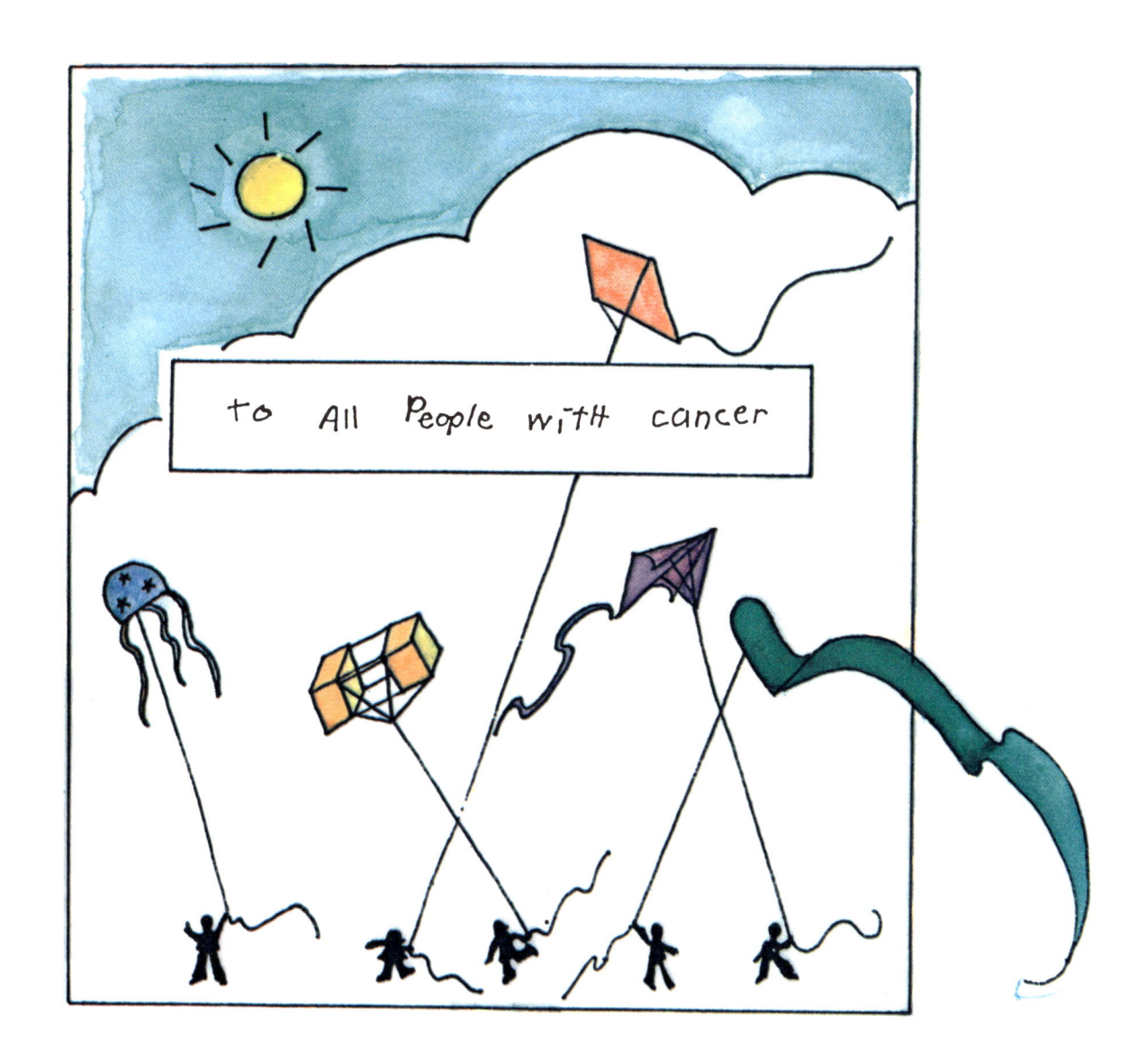

CANCER IS THE pits!

Page 1

CHAPTer 1: WHAT Happend

MY NAME IS MATTHEW LANCaster I AM 10 YEAR'S OLD, I Live in NORTH CANTON, OHio. WHEN I WAS 9 YEAR'S OLD. I WAS Visiting MY GRAND Parents in ALABAMA, AND I STARTED HAVing PAIN In MY LEFT Leg. WHen I got BAck TO OHio I WENT TO See My ORTHipeDic Doctor Dr. KANG, He SAiD TO GO to tHE HospitAL. SO I went to timken Murcey MEDicaL center. I HAD to Have AN Operation, tHey Removed Some tissu. AND THEN I WAS DiAgnosed AS A Uing SarcomA PacItint. I WAS very ScareD, I DiDinT Even Now WHAT A Uing SarcomA tomer was. It WAS in My LEFT Leg By tHE FiBULA. I WAS in tHE HospitAL for About A Week AND A HALF. WHen I Left I WAS on CRuttes for A Month. MY MoTHer toLD ME I WouLD HAVE TO GO to A DocTor in Akron Every THREWEEKS. I DiDent think that Was THAT BAD.

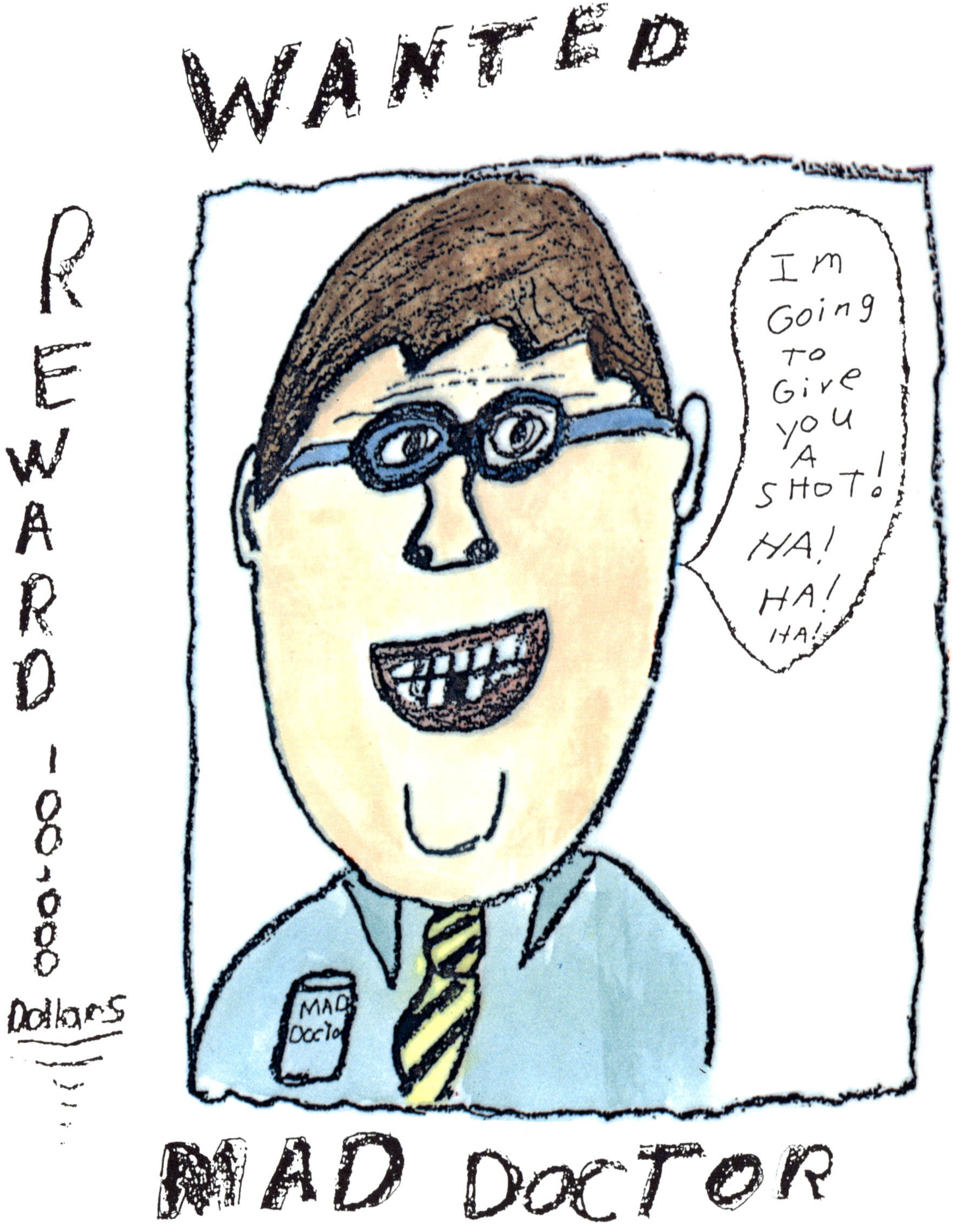
WANTED
REWARD 100,000 Dollars
Im Going to Give you A SHOT! HA! HA! HA!
MAD Doctor
MAD DOCTOR

Page 2

I FELT Like it wasn't FAir why me, But THen I ReLized How many Pepol in tHE world Have Cancer. But You Just Have to HAng on! Grit Your teeTH, Have A positive Attatude, You can Do AnytHing You set Your mind to. Keep telling YourseLF you can Do iT!

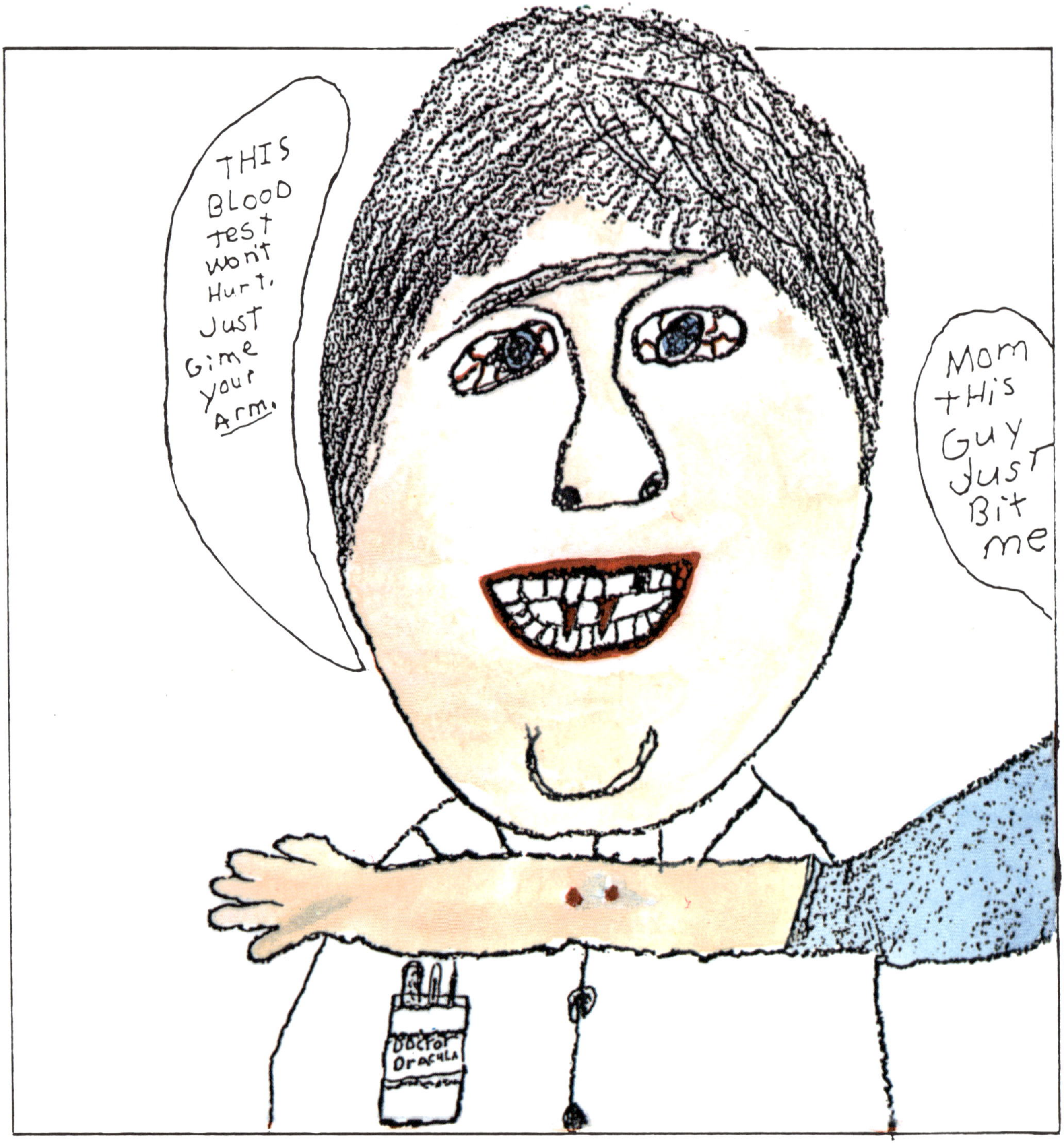
THIS BLOOD Test won't Hurt. Just Gime your Arm.
Mom this Guy Just Bit me
Doctor Dracula

CHAPTER 2   Page 3

Kymo Therpy

THE First time I went to AKRon CHiLDRens HospitAL, I Saw A Doctor NAMED DR. KAstLik HE SAiD tHAt I WOULD Have to Have MEDAcation, tHAt onLy Can Be given By injection, AnD PiLLS, AnD I Like evry otHer KiD I HatE SHoots, AnD PiLL's. THE MeDAcation's Name's where Sytoxin, ADRAMiAcen, VencHristin, DeActomiAcel Sytoxin is An I.V. (in Vane), tHE Rest ARe SHoots. Sytoxin made me Sick For A Day, ADRAMiAcen made me Sick For A Hour or two. VENcHristin DiDn't make me sick. But wHen you get sick Just tHink it will BE OVER Soon Don't tHink ABout it. TAKE Your minD of it. WHen you tAke Pill's Just Say to Yourself You can Do it, WASH it Down witH Some Liquid, AND BE tHANKFull it's not A sHoot! HAVE A Positive ADituD. AND if tHere ReaL Big see if you can Put tHem crusHuD up in Juice AnD DRink it!

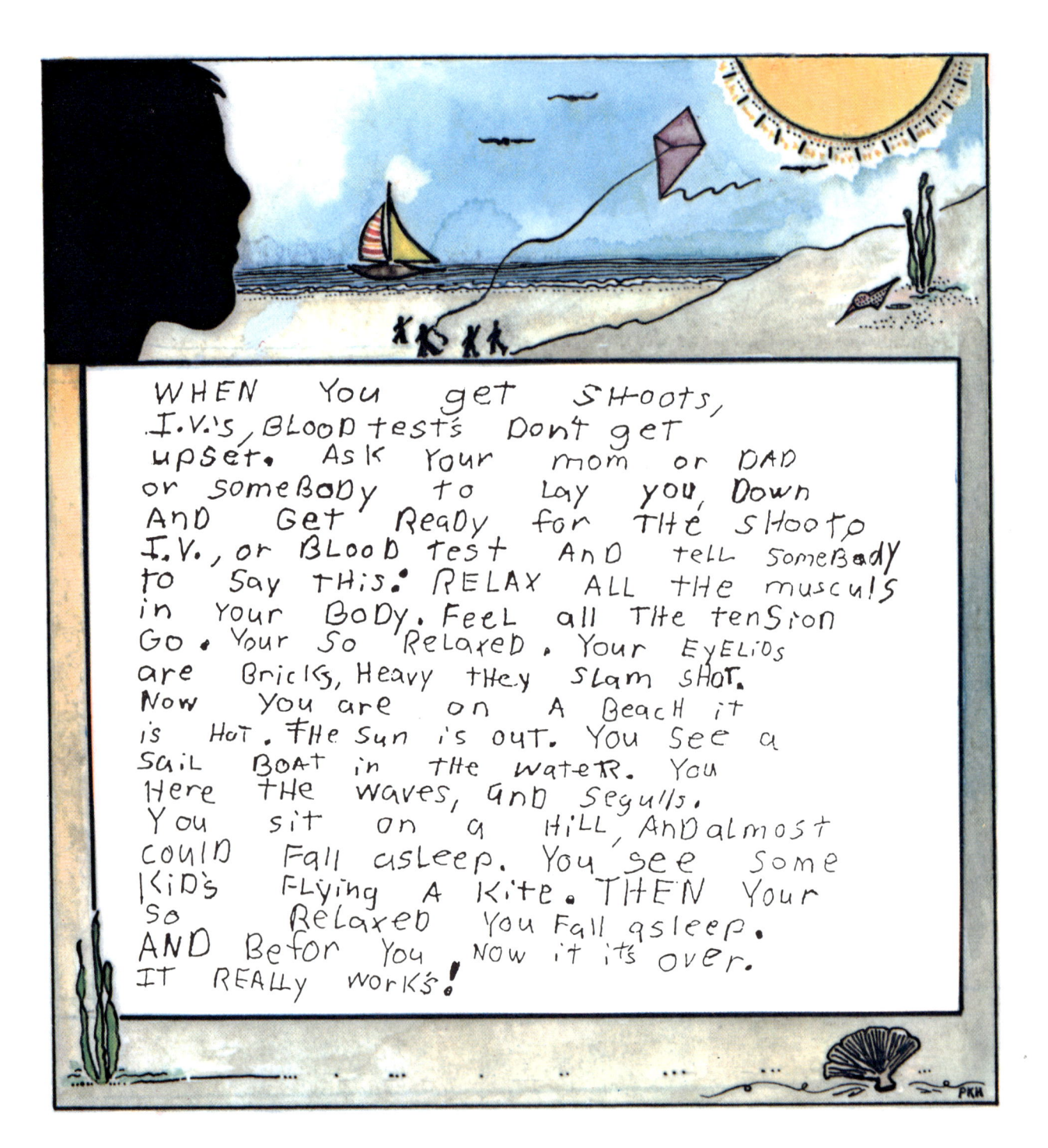

WHEN You get SHoots, I.V.'s, BLooD tests Don't get upset. Ask Your mom or DAD or someBoDy to Lay you Down AnD Get ReaDy for THe sHoot o I.V., or BLooD test AnD tell someBody to say tHis: RELAX ALL tHe musculs in Your BoDy. FeeL all THe tenSion Go. Your So Relaxed. Your EyeLiDs are Bricks, Heavy tHey sLam SHot. Now you are on A Beach it is Hot. tHe Sun is out. You See a SaiL BoAt in tHe wateR. You Here tHe waves, anD Segulls. You sit on a HiLL, AnD almost couLD Fall asleep. You see some KiDs FLying A kite. THEN Your so Relaxed You Fall asleep. AND Befor You Now it it's over. IT REALLy works!

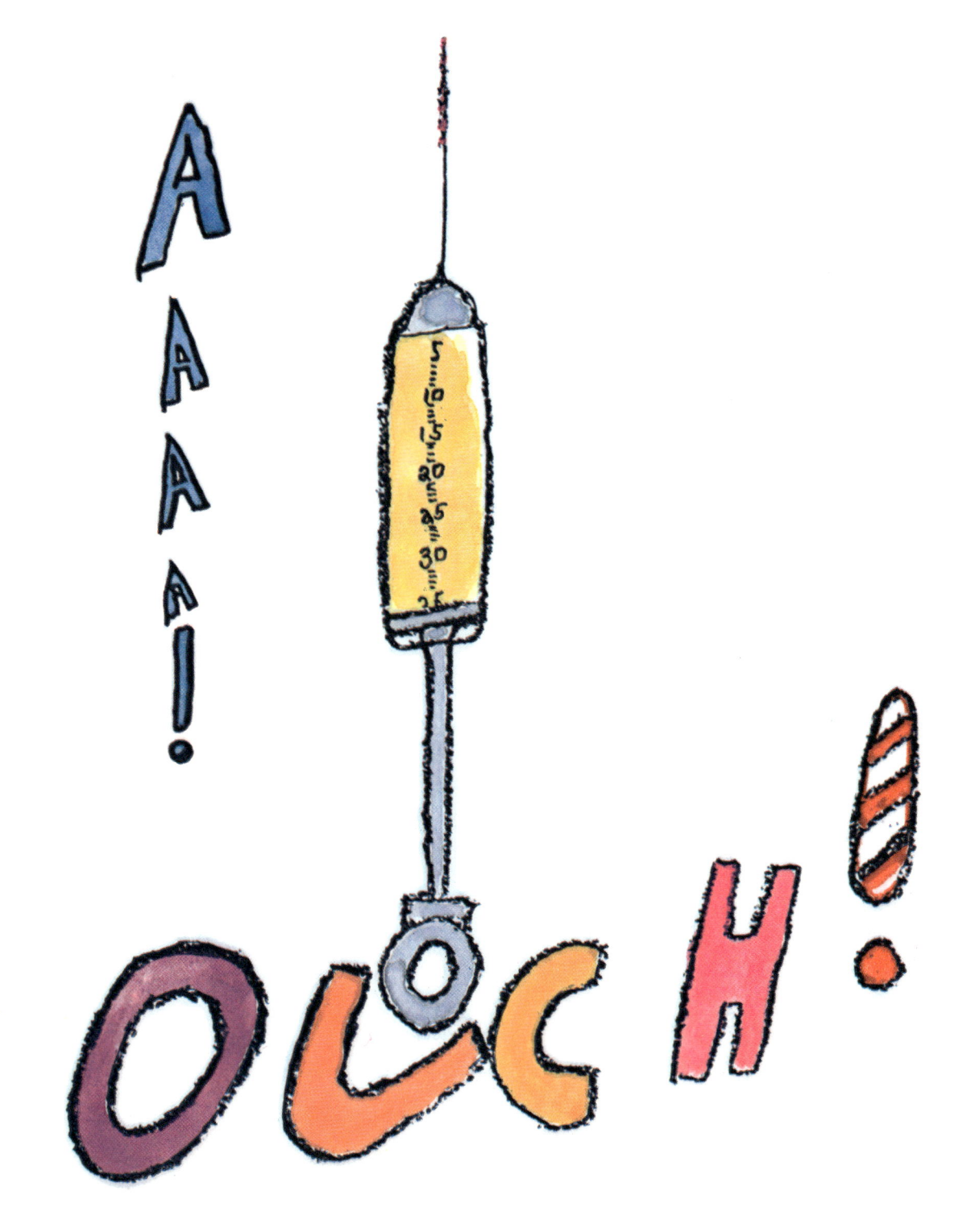

Chapter 3   Page 5

Radiation

I have had to have radiation 4 times six weeks on my leg, six weeks on my spine, five days on my neck, ten weeks on my verbabra. If you have to take Flagil crush it up put it in grape juice! Radiation is pretty easy, just hold still. It is like a laser from Star Wars!

CHAPTER 4   PAGE 6

I FEEL THIS WAY

I HAVE HAD TO HAV KYMO THERAPY For A Year. It Has Been Very Hard. I'v Been in A Hospital 3 times in the Last Year. Hospitals are Fun for 3 or 4 Days, But I Stayed in for 3 Weeks only 2 of the times. When I was 9 I Thoght I Was THE Only one and THAT it wasn't fair, AnD it is not But it Happend, AND You And I Have to Except it. I'm sure You FELT THE Same. I Was Scrard. VERY Scard. I Have HAD more THan one tomor, 2 more, 1 in my Neck, 1 on my spine. AND some Broke. AS You NOW the spine Has Nerves on it. I Hav Not Been ABLe to walk for 3 months. But if I Can Handle it You can! I Have Lost my Hair, You mite to But it will come Back. mine is! IF Your friends Laght AT You THE Not very Good FRIENDS.

Chapter 5 — Page 7

IF YOU CAN'T WALK.

IF YOU can't walk your not ALONE. I can't. I FELT Like I was the AnLy ONE, BuT I Recently went to WALT Disny world, AND I Relized How many Pepol can't walk. I THoght I would Be able to walk By CHritmas, But I, Didn't. BuT, I Havent Given up. I'm Scard, it's Been 3 months. So Just Hang on. Tell Yourself it Hasen't Happend yet, But it will! IF you ARE Mad, scard, Afraid TALK to Someone. Dont Give UP, Never! I'm very scard, I THink it would Be HoriBal not To WALK. But I Never Give up. I Now I Miss school, And wHat Really Makes me MAD is I can't Do tHings myself Like turn off the TV, Easy THings.

Chapter 6   Page 8

PAIN

WHEN You Have cancer you Experenc A LoT of Pain, But you wiLL Hav to Bare it. Just say it wiLL Be over soon. Don't Panic, Grit your teeth and Before you Now it it wiLL Be over. TAKE Deep Breths. Just Relax.

Chapter 7   page 9

MEDiCTiON

I HAVE HaD six Difrent MEDicons CoDin, Volume, PREDNazon, FLagiL, tafarin, septru WHen you take mebicins Just put it in tHE Back of your MouTH SwaLLo WasH witH water. Don't cik yourself up. Becaus you will tHrow it up. Say you CAN Get it Down in your stomac, tHen EAT SomeTHing AND THEN it's over.

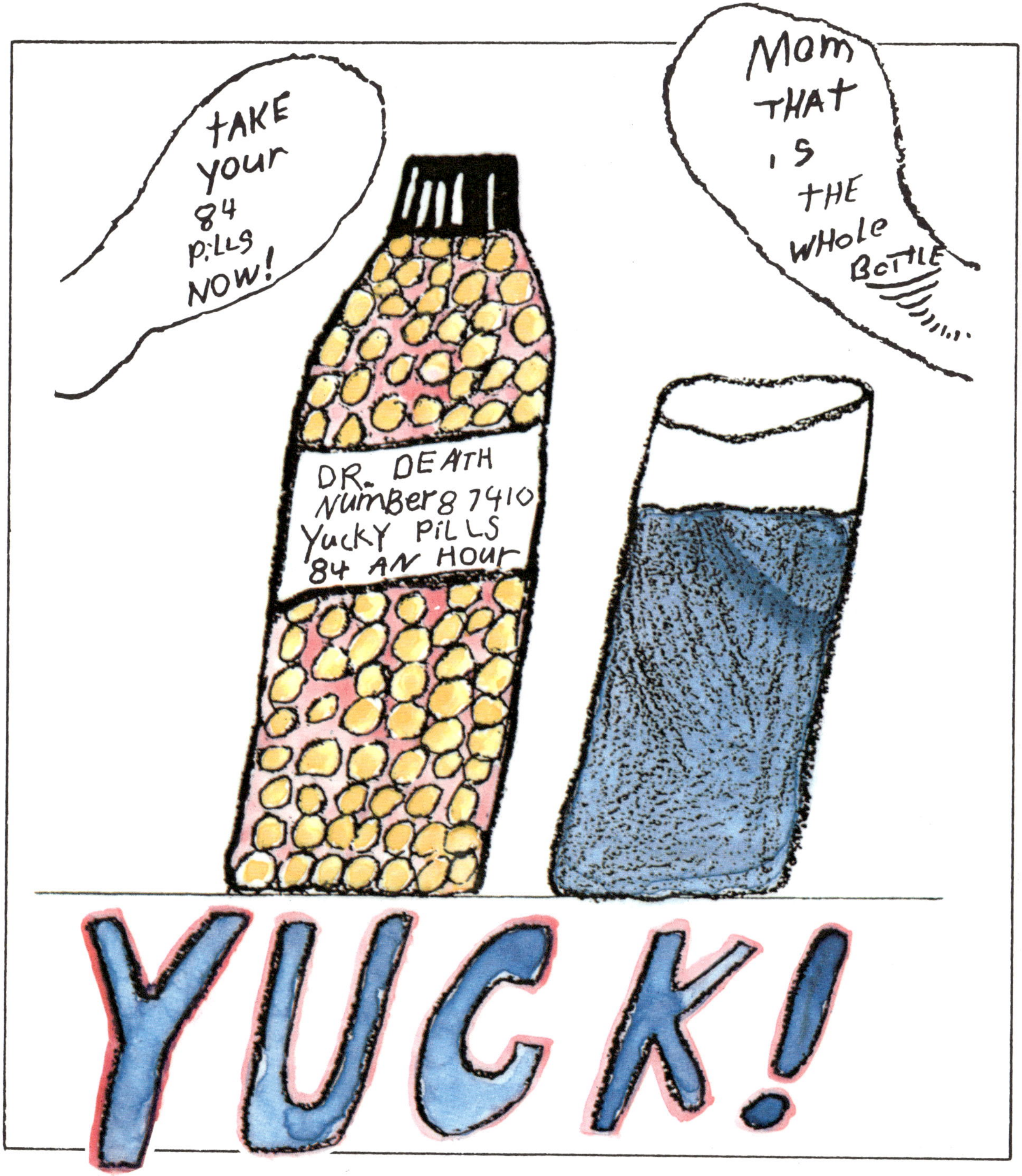
take your 84 pills NOW!
Mom THAT is THE WHOLE BOTTLE
DR. DEATH
Number 8 7410
Yucky PiLLS
84 AN Hour
YUCK!

Chapter 8　　　　　　　　　　　　　　　　　　　Page 10

Scary DREAMS

I Now I Have HaD A Lot of Scary tHogHts, You PRoBaLe DO to. I THink Before I Go to tHe Doctor, Will He Put me in tHE Hospital? WiLL He give me A sHot? WiLL He Hurt me? Will He tell me I'm not going to walk? WHen You get tHogHts Like tHAT, PuT tHem out of Your minD, THink ABouT Something ELSe. AnyTHing ELSe. AND Be Happy.

THE NIGHT NURSES......

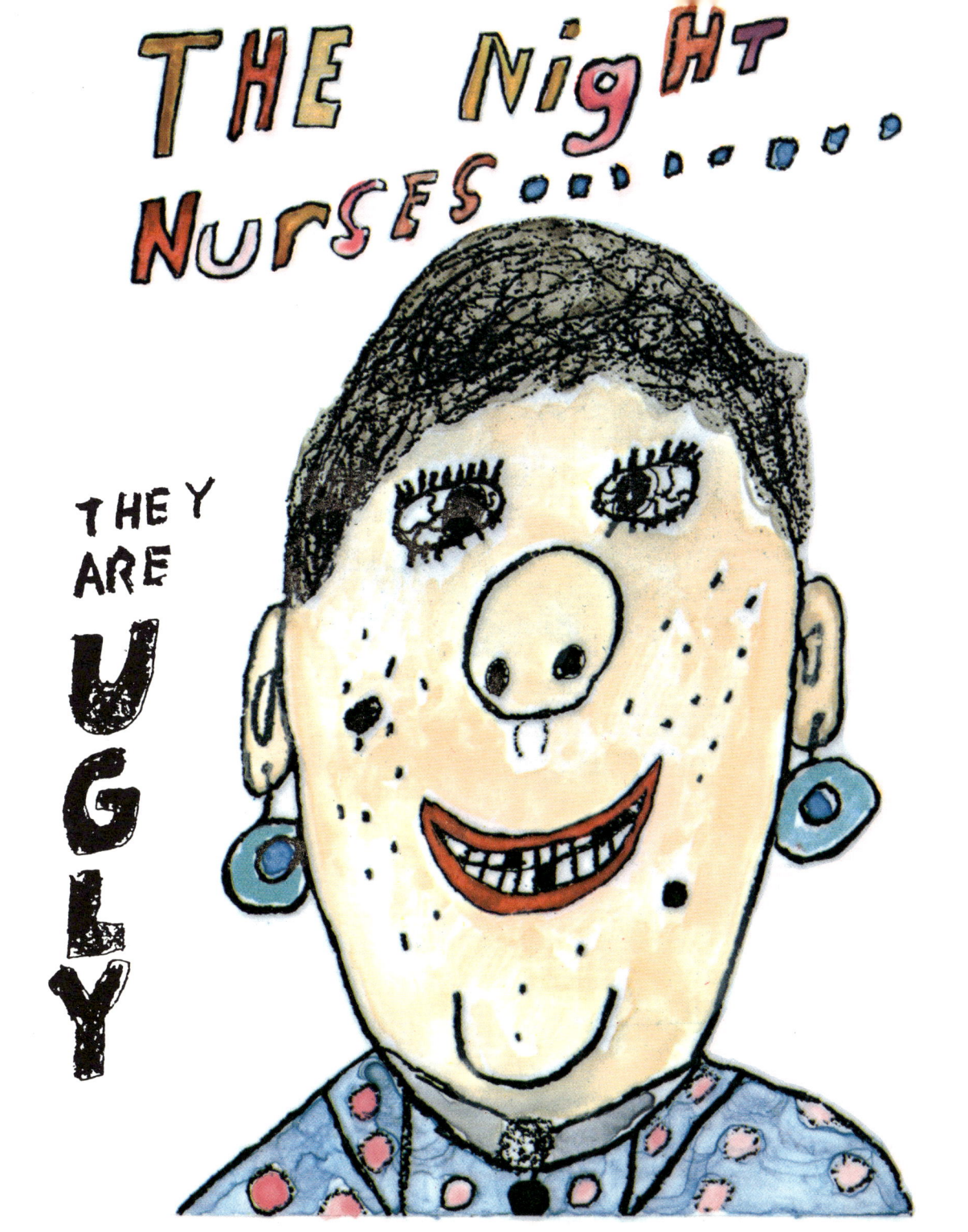

THEY ARE UGLY

Chapter 9   Page 11

IT'S NOT Fair

Is it Fair THAT it HappenD to you AND I? NO! But it DiD AnD We Hav to ExsepT it. AND KEEP on Hanging in tHER. Don't Give up. You can DO Anything you set Your minD to. I THoghT I WAS THE ONLY one in tHE World, AND THAT IT wasn't Fair, AND is not Fair. You Have TO Be PaSanT. My Doctor sa THAT I mite stop Kymo tHerpy, AnD if I can StanDit YOU CAN!

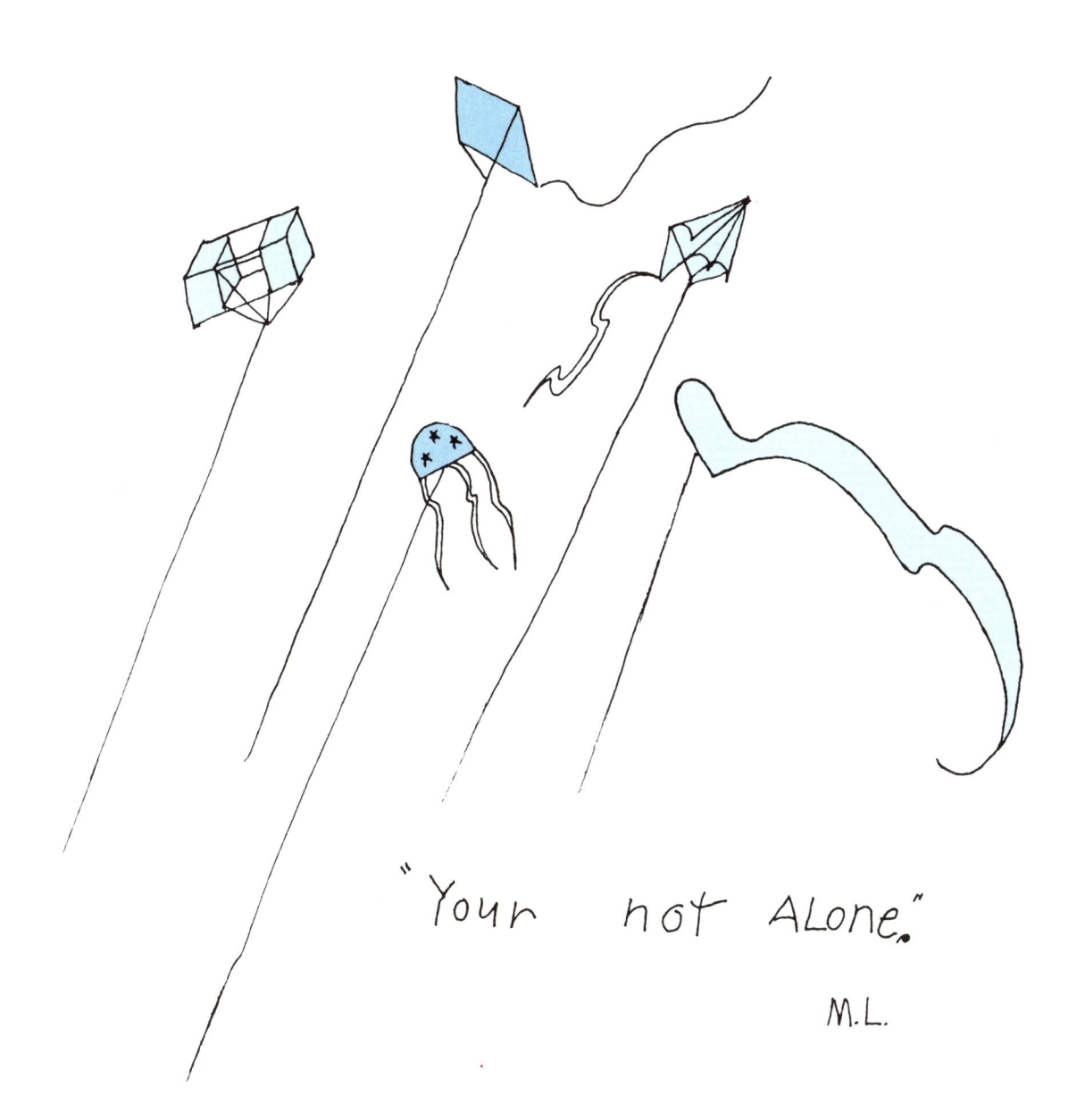

"Your not Alone."

M.L.

Chapter 10   Page 12

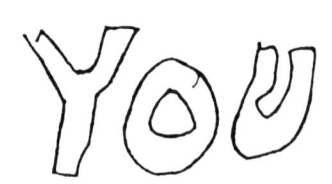

YOU

I know that you will be able to handle cancer. Becaus if I can you can. It's O.K. to be scard. You hav to hav a positiv aditud. Say to yourself you can do anything. Never say you can't. You just hav to hang in ther. I think you can do it. I rote this book to help people with cancer, your not alone.

HANG TOUGHF

I Dont know if you are very Religis, But RemBer in tHE BiBLE WHEN Jesus HealD tHE BLinD MAN in a seconD, Well HE wiLL Do tHE same for you, EVEN if it TAKE'S A MontH or A Year, He **WiLL!** I Have Recently Been in tHE Hospital Again! to tRy New MEDiceny I tHougHt tHAT WHAT I HAD WAS tHE wours! But my two RoomAts, ONE HADE AN ACCiDent wHen HE WAS DRiving in His car A tRuck Hit tHE Top of tHE CAR BRoke His Back, HE WAS in tHE Hospital in NocomA For 5½ montHs. WHEN HE came out HE HAD to Learn to tALk Again, How To Get DResseD again. AnD HE was Paralized from tHE miDDle of tHE CHEST Down, for Life. AND YEt He StiLL is Happy At First I tHougt He HaD A NomonyA. tHE OTHER WAS RetarDeD FRom BirtHt, But He Was still HAPPy AnD if WE Can Do it You can to.!

on Back

AND RemeBer Hang tougHf, PositiY ADituD, ALL THE Time. AND PRAY to GoD.